The McMillin Method:

How to Self-Treat Chronic Dizziness and PPPD Workbook

By: Amy McMillin, PT
Vestibular Physical Therapist

The McMillin Method:

How to Self-Treat Chronic Dizziness and PPPD Workbook

This Workbook Belongs To:

_____

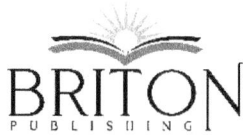

BRITON
PUBLISHING

Briton Publishing, LLC
810 Eastgate North Dr., Suite 200
Cincinnati, Ohio 45245
www.britonpublishing.com

ISBN: 978-1-956216-17-2

Briton Publishing books are distributed by Ingram Content Group and made available worldwide.

CONTENTS

DISCLAIMER

I am a licensed physical therapist; however, please be aware that I am not *your* physical therapist. It is crucial to understand that any questions you have should be directed to your healthcare provider, as the information provided here is for general purposes only.

The content provided in this medical workbook is intended for informational and educational purposes only. It is not a substitute for professional medical advice, diagnosis, or treatment. Always seek the advice of your physician or other qualified health provider with any questions you may have regarding a medical condition.

This workbook is designed to complement, not replace, the relationship that exists between a patient and their healthcare provider. The exercises, activities, and information contained herein are not exhaustive and may not be suitable for everyone. Individual health conditions and requirements vary, and it is imperative to consult with a qualified healthcare professional before implementing any recommendations in this workbook.

The author and publisher disclaim responsibility for any adverse effects or consequences resulting directly or indirectly from the use of the information provided in this workbook. No guarantees or assurances are made regarding specific outcomes or results based on the use of this workbook.

The information, exercises, and techniques presented are based on general medical knowledge available at the time of writing and are subject to change. The author and publisher do not endorse any specific products, services, or organizations mentioned in this workbook.

By using this workbook, you agree to release and hold harmless the author, publisher, and any contributors from any and all claims, liabilities, or damages arising from your use of the information provided herein.

This disclaimer is subject to change without notice, and users are encouraged to review it regularly for any updates.

Please refrain from using this content for self-diagnosis or self-treatment of any health, medical, or physical conditions. By accessing and utilizing this content, you agree to hold harmless and indemnify Custom Care Rehab, LLC, and its owner/employees from any losses, injuries, or damages resulting from claims arising out of your use or misuse of this information.

It is important to note that the outcomes of educational content or recommendations provided on the company's website, social media, products, blog, email series, and workbooks cannot be guaranteed. Any comments or suggestions made by Custom Care Rehab, LLC, and its owner, Amy McMillin, are expressions of opinion and should not be considered absolute advice.

INTRODUCTION

Have you ever felt your world spinning out of control, your every step marred by persistent dizziness? In these moments, it's easy to lose sight of your strength, but I'm here to guide you through a transformative journey of healing. Welcome, to the next part of your journey in self-recovery from chronic dizziness. This workbook is designed to provide you with a comprehensive approach to managing and conquering chronic dizziness through the powerful framework of Vestibular Therapy with a Cognitive Behavioral Therapy (CBT) approach. This guide is uniquely designed to be self-paced and focused on function over symptoms.

Whether you're experiencing frequent bouts of dizziness or struggling with persistent feelings of imbalance, this workbook is tailored to help you regain control over your body's response to dizziness and improve your overall quality of life. Dizziness can significantly impact your daily activities, from work to leisure and even simple tasks can become challenging.

This step-by-step guide is crafted to empower you with the necessary tools, exercises, and insights to navigate through the complexities of chronic dizziness. With dedicated commitment and the guidance provided in these pages, you can make significant strides towards overcoming dizziness and reclaiming your body again.

I commend you for taking this important step toward improving your well-being and invite you to embark on this journey with me. Remember, every step you take brings you closer to a life free from the constraints of chronic dizziness.

Best wishes on your path to steadiness and well-being,

—*Amy McMillin, Vestibular Physical Therapist*

DEFINING PERSISTENT POSTURAL PERCEPTUAL DIZZINESS

Before delving into the details of treatment, let's establish a clear understanding of 3PD, its characteristics, and the diagnostic process. PPPD, or 3PD, previously known as chronic subjective dizziness, has characteristics of non-vertiginous, or non-spinning, dizziness and fluctuating unsteadiness provoked by visual stimuli that cannot be explained by another vestibular disorder.

3PD is diagnosed through exclusion and no laboratory tests can definitively confirm. However, one may confirm an underlying diagnosis that may have led to the subsequent 3PD symptoms. It is typically triggered shortly after a true vestibular event that causes a disruption of balance like benign paroxysmal positional vertigo, vestibular neuritis, Meniere's disease, stroke, vestibular migraine, concussion, whiplash, or panic attack with dizziness.

Presentation and history include:

- Unsteadiness, imbalance, or non-spinning dizziness

- Present for 3 months or longer

- Fluctuating severity

- Triggers can include intense visual tasks like reading, crowds, shopping stores, computer work, action television, busy airports, or restaurants

- Can also be provoked by moving yourself in your environment

The mechanism of causing symptoms is not fully understood. Following a vestibular incident, or even a panic attack with dizziness, it is hypothesized that a person has changes in reliance on visual cues for balance and becomes hypervigilant regarding their environment. One relies heavily on vision instead of the vestibular or touch systems for balance. This leads to symptoms when a person is moving and when in visually demanding environments like airports, casinos, or grocery stores. Behavioral co-morbidities like obsessive-compulsive disorder, mild depression, and anxiety may contribute to developing 3PD. Physical symptoms of unsteadiness and dizziness can lead to frustration and avoidance of activities that cause symptoms. This causes a vicious cycle of tolerating less and less stimulation or movement.

The following section outlines various treatments for 3PD. However, it's crucial to consult with a healthcare professional to determine the most suitable approach for your individual needs. Treatment recommendations include[1]:

- Vestibular Rehabilitation Therapy (VRT), which includes cognitive behavioral therapy techniques in my approach.
- Medication, SSRIs (selective serotonin reuptake inhibitors) or SNRIs (serotonin norepinephrine reuptake inhibitors). Pharmaceutical treatment is very slowly introduced and suggested to be maintained for at least a year to minimize the chance of relapse, prescribed by a physician[2].

- Cognitive Behavioral Therapy with a certified therapist to talk through the emotional aspect of suffering from chronic dizziness.

This workbook will primarily discuss vestibular rehab therapy, as it is the technique I can speak to professionally and within the scope of my license. If you haven't consulted a licensed vestibular therapist, it's highly recommended to do so. Individualized treatment plans are essential, and a professional can guide you through the most suitable approach for your situation. With that being said, not all people can obtain access to a vestibular specialist well-versed in the treatment of 3PD. In addition, not all vestibular therapists are created the same. Some have an advanced understanding of the disorder, and some do not. I have seen many clients who have tried vestibular therapy only to be given bad information or simply an incomplete plan of care that leads to the failure of their vestibular rehab.

The McMillin Method for the treatment of 3PD uses 5 principles:

1) Cardiovascular Exercise

2) Gaze Stability

3) Grounding Balance Exercises

4) Nervous System Regulation

5) Habituation
   - Visual Based
   - Self-Movement Based

This structured program, backed by the latest research, offers a self-paced journey for managing 3PD symptoms effectively. Using a unique blend of evidence-based methods and cognitive behavioral therapy techniques, we shift focus from symptoms to function. This workbook serves as a practical guide, ensuring an organized and easy-to-follow home exercise program. By reframing your mindset and measuring progress through daily activities, rather than symptom intensity, we aim for a fuller recovery and a better quality of life. Experience the power of combining vestibular therapy with behavioral changes for lasting results.

REFLECTION

My initial vertigo occurred on this date:

_____

What were my physical limitations the first 3 months after my vertigo occurrence?

_____

_____

_____

_____

_____

_____

_____

_____

_____

_____

_____

_____

_____

_____

_____

_____

_____

_____

My Remaining Functional Limitations Include:

An example might be, "I cannot stay in a Costco for more than 5 minutes. I cannot turn my head when walking. I cannot sit in a restaurant. I still get dizzy putting my shoes on."

_____

_____

_____

_____

_____

_____

Date:_____

My Current Symptoms Include:

Please Rank the Intensity of your Symptoms (0-10/10) (0 Being None, 10 Being Most Intense)

_____

_____

_____

_____

_____

_____

_____

_____

_____

_____

_____

_____

The reason I wanted you to reflect on the initial injury is to realize how far you have already come. You suffered a physical trauma that significantly altered your life's course. However, there is more to you than a physical impairment. You are more than your dizziness; it is a part of your experience, not the totality of your being. I like the thought… dizziness is a part of you but it does not define all of you.

As you embark on this healing journey from chronic dizziness, I encourage you to embrace and nurture every aspect of yourself. While dizziness and its symptoms may be present, they need not dominate your entire existence. In my experience, the most remarkable recoveries from chronic dizziness occur when individuals can shift their focus to their positive attributes, accepting their current circumstances while also acknowledging their resilience and inner strength.

Your journey toward recovery is as much about reclaiming your sense of self-worth and resilience as it is about managing the physical symptoms. By nurturing a holistic view of yourself and your capabilities, you can cultivate a mindset that empowers you to confront challenges and discover newfound inner resources. Hopefully, this resonates and speaks to some of the emotions you have felt. However, now I want you to be more excited for what is to come!

This workbook will focus on the treatment of 3PD, as it is the most common cause of chronic dizziness. I am passionate about this topic because chronic dizziness CAN be treated, there is a method to follow, and I want to spread the word far and wide!

Having helped countless patients throughout my career, I understand the overwhelming challenges it presents. I have seen people at their absolute worst. Some patients with ten years of chronic dizziness without answers from the medical community, are withdrawn from their friends and families and confined to their homes. Other patients have control over their symptoms within two to three months of onset but struggle with flare-ups of dizziness during stressful times in their lives. The journey isn't just about overcoming symptoms; it's about rediscovering your resilience and reclaiming your life.

It is important to stress that there is no 100% cure for 3PD and everyone's journey is individualized. One's outcomes will depend on the initial diagnosis, the care you received up to now, and your level of readiness to accept any amount of "win" you accomplish. It is important to remember treatment goals are to improve function, experience the least amount of symptoms, and have a better quality of life.

This workbook is more than just a guide—it's a companion on your path to overcoming chronic dizziness. Through practical exercises, insights, and evidence-based strategies, we'll navigate the complexities of 3PD together, unlocking a future where dizziness no longer defines your days. My method of treatment is rooted in evidence-based research and will highlight the currently recommended treatment approaches in 3PD. I invite you to actively engage with the exercises and insights provided in this workbook, as they are designed to be your companions on the path to recovery.

SETTING UP FOR SUCCESS

Before you begin the vestibular therapy portion of this workbook, I want to address the current evidence-based treatment approach. Currently, the research indicates that the three-pronged approach of vestibular therapy, cognitive behavioral therapy, and anti-depressant medication gives a person the best rate of recovery. However, as with everything in medicine, this is just a recommendation. I have had patients who have side effects with every type of medication the doctor throws their way. I have had patients who do not wish to try medications and opt for a holistic approach. I have had patients who can only start vestibular therapy after medication has been introduced for three months, and only then do they tolerate vestibular rehab. I have had patients who need to go to cognitive behavioral therapy to talk through trauma or talk through the anxiety of being chronically dizzy before they can start vestibular therapy. I have had patients who only follow my therapy approach and do not need medication or cognitive behavioral therapy.

My point in telling you these anecdotes is that everyone's journey is different and individualized. There is no right way to begin and unfortunately, there is no exact timeline. Some people feel better in two weeks; some people feel improvement in months. You just need to try a path and pivot if needed. If you decide to start with the vestibular therapy approach first and find that symptoms are simply too elevated, try medication or counseling first. Then come back to the workbook at a later date.

It is important to know, that there is not a single person who has not benefited in some way from my treatment approach. You may not get full relief from your symptoms, but I can promise you more good days than bad, an increase in your function, and coping mechanisms to manage your dizziness. Start your recovery with those intentions and you will have success!

SELF-TREAT YOUR DIZZINESS

The following chapters will detail the treatment protocol I use with my clients who suffer from chronic dizziness and PPPD. I would like to begin with an outline of the general prescription I give to my clients; however, these are goals to work up to. Every person reaches these exercise goals at their own pace. Just do what you can without causing symptoms to flare up and stay elevated for longer than 30 minutes. If you try to exercise and your symptoms elevate, please do less and slowly add repetitions or minutes as able until you reach the desired goals.

EXERCISE PLAN

1) Cardiovascular workout 150 minutes per week

2) 20 minutes of gaze stability exercises 4-5 days per week

3) 20 minutes of grounding and balance exercises 4-5 days per week

4) Meditation or relaxation exercises 5 minutes daily, minimum

5) Habituation exercises 5 reps daily of 1-2 tasks until 0-1/10 dizzy experienced in said task

Cardiovascular Exercise

Why is cardiovascular exercise my first treatment strategy? It is an important part of healing from 3PD! I am not just loosely encouraging you to work out more; there is real evidence in the research supporting the effectiveness of using exercise to heal your brain.

It is very similar to the physiologic reason people who suffer concussions or strokes are treated with cardio exercise and blood perfusion. Blood perfusion is the act of promoting blood flow to the brain. Moderate to high-intensity cardio exercise allows for the heart to start pumping and pushing blood up toward the brain.

As we get blood to the brain, it brings with it oxygen and important neurotransmitters like serotonin, dopamine, and norepinephrine. Neurotransmitters are chemical messengers in the body that allow us to do everything we do, think, and feel!

I commonly speak in analogies. This is how I explain neurotransmitters to my clients, "Imagine our brain is a cake. We need the right amount of ingredients to make our cake taste right, feel right, and bake correctly. For example, say you made your cake with one tablespoon of sugar instead of one cup of sugar we still have a cake, but it will not taste right. That one ingredient blunder will ruin your cake. The same issue happens in our brains. If our ingredients, aka our neurotransmitters, are at the wrong levels our bodies do not function correctly."

One may experience symptoms like brain fog, dizziness, memory issues, balance issues, rapid heart rate, sleeplessness, depression, anxiety, muscle fatigue, and so much more.

With cardiovascular exercise you can normalize your neurotransmitters, thus leading to decreasing the symptoms listed above.

The second reason behind adding cardio exercise into the treatment protocol for PPPD is neuroplasticity. Neuroplasticity is the ability of the brain and nerves to grow. The brain and its neural network are always learning new things, adapting to challenges, and evolving to stress. Cardio exercise allows for greater potential for growth by "prepping" the brain with more blood flow and neurotransmitters. I recommend starting your vestibular rehab program with twenty to twenty-five minutes of cardio exercise and then trying your gaze stability exercises.

You may find that your gaze stability exercises are more tolerable and more effective when doing cardio first. Exercise can also calm your sympathetic nervous system, which is responsible for the "fight or flight" response, thus making you less anxious when completing your vestibular therapy.

Exercise Plan

Research suggests that 150 minutes a week of various types of exercise including brisk walking, lifting weights, or cycling at moderate to high intensity is beneficial for mental health and physical health [3].

Here is how we calculate moderate to high intensity:

First, what is your resting heart rate: _____(a).

Second, take (220-age) =_____ (b)

Third, take (b-a): _____ (c)

Next, multiply (c) by x .60 (d). Then add the resting heart rate (a) back in. This is your moderate-intensity goal. Repeat the process with .80 for your high-intensity goal. Do not worry, I will go through an example next.

Example: My resting heart rate is 72 (a). My age is 41.

$220 - 41 = 179$ (b)

$(b - a) = 107$ (c)

$107 \times .60 = 64.2$ (d)

$(d + a)$ $64.2 + 72 = \textbf{136.2}$

Repeating the process for high intensity or 80% is: $107 \times .80 = 85.6$

$85.6 + 72 = \textbf{157.6}$

So, my heart rate goal is *136.2 to 157.6* for 150 minutes a week. Now your turn!

Resting heart rate is _____ (a)

Age is _____

$220 - age =$ _____ (b)

$(b - a) =$ _____ (c)

(c) _____ x .60 = _____ (d)

(d) + (a) = _____

Repeating the process for high intensity or 80%: _____

Heart rate goals: _____

Remember this is a goal to work towards you should not start at this heart rate goal for 150 minutes right away. Pace yourself and enjoy the process of trying to achieve it. If you are on medication that slows your heart rate this formula may not apply to you. In that case, use a self-assessment 0-10/10 scale. Try to aim for a 5-7/10 scale, with 10 being as hard as you can go.

Always consult a physician before starting any new cardiovascular routine.

Gaze Stability

Gaze Stability exercises are the foundation of vestibular therapy. They are specific exercises to strengthen inner ear nerve weakness and the balance centers of the brain. They are known as gaze stability, vestibular adaptation, or Vestibulo-Ocular Reflex, VOR, exercises. The whole function of the vestibular system is to sense your direction and to keep your eyes stable as you walk, run, or move. If your vestibular system has been impaired you will feel off balance, dizzy, or have blurry vision when you move about. Gaze stability exercises are meant to improve the ability of your inner ear to keep your eyes steady and stay balanced.

If your initial cause of vertigo was diagnosed as a vestibular hypofunction, gaze stability exercises should be a definite part of your recovery plan. Vestibular hypofunction is a medical term used to describe weakness in one or both vestibular nerves. This can happen with a viral attack, Covid-19, chronic Meniere's disease, concussion, or a tumor on the nerve. I also prescribe gaze stability exercises to any person who has a dizziness level of 2/10 or more when testing VOR x 1 exercises. If you need gaze stability exercises you will feel dizzy during them!

I will include my general exercises and progressions on the next page, but you may find it useful to visit my YouTube page, *Treat Dizziness at Home*, for video demonstrations of gaze stability exercises. Gaze stability exercises should be performed at least twelve to twenty minutes a day[4] however, they do not have to be performed continuously. You can do one exercise at a time and go back to complete another exercise later in the day.

The purpose of these exercises is to preserve any function of the vestibular nerve, reinforce when the vestibular system should be active, and habituate to movement; which is so commonly avoided with 3PD. During gaze stability exercises, you shake your head small and quickly; trying to move the head as quickly as possible while keeping the image clear. These exercises will make your dizziness increase but only temporarily. Our goal is *not* to increase symptoms by more than just a few points on a 0-10/10 scale. However, you may feel tired from exercise; this is common. Keep in mind dizziness from exercise is common but should be resolved back to baseline within 15 minutes.

Home Exercise Program

VOR x 1 Near: Hold a pencil, shake your head small but quickly while keeping your eyes locked onto the eraser of the pencil. **Left and Right, Up and Down x 60 seconds each.**

VOR x 1 Far: look at "x" on wall or object across the room. Shake your head small but quickly while keeping your gaze locked onto the target. **Left and Right, Up and Down x 60 seconds each.**

VOR x 2: head and pencil move opposite of one another. **60 seconds left and right. Repeat up and down.**

Gaze Stability: read the "letter page" (Appendix 1), small but quick. Reading one letter at a time, completing the whole page. **Keep the head moving, but the letter stays clear while reading.**

Imaginary VOR: eyes on target, close eyes & move head 45 degrees to the right. Open your eyes and your eyes should stay on the initial target to the left. **Repeat up and down. 30 seconds each way.**

Two Target Eye Shift: move eyes to target then head, repeat to other side. You can vary the speed and direction of the target. **Perform 1-2 minutes in different directions.**

Now when doing these exercises if you find that your dizziness makes you worse for longer than 15 minutes you must modify it. Every exercise is modifiable! You can decrease your time or repetitions until you can tolerate an exercise without causing lingering dizziness.

You can move your head slower during exercise and increase speed as you feel able. Some clients need to start in a comfortable seated position to complete the exercises until they can tolerate progressing to standing or walking. Below are the recommended progressions of the exercise program. Remember your goal is to complete each exercise without increasing dizziness past a 0-2/10 scale. Once this is achieved you can progress to the next challenge. Your end goal is to be able to complete the exercise without dizziness, walking, and at normal speed.

Exercise progression is as follows:

Seated

Standing

Foam pad/pillow

Walking

Outdoor walking

Use of backgrounds:

Blank background

Busy background, like patterned wallpaper

Use of a busy visual target, like a checkerboard

Each stage should be completed with a blank and then a busy background. Proceed to the next stage only when all exercises can be completed with dizziness of 0-2/10 intensity levels.

Grounding and Balance

Grounding refers to a state of body awareness and connection with the supporting surface or floor. It involves a conscious and intentional focus on the body's sensory input, emphasizing stability, balance, and a sense of being rooted. Overall, being grounded is a heightened awareness of one's body to its ground, promoting stability, balance, and a mindful connection with the present moment. Oftentimes, I will ask my clients to "pay attention to what your feet are telling you." If one can ground, one can combat the dizziness.

With 3PD visual dizziness is quite common. When the inner ear cannot be relied upon to provide accurate information, one may start to become dependent on the visual system. The problem with this compensatory strategy is that when the brain experiences a visually moving environment it cannot tell if the body is still or moving. The brain has difficulty sensing that the visual environment is moving but the body can remain still. One example would be watching action television. When a person is seated but watching a movie that has someone run across the screen, someone with visual dependence may feel like they are moving!

Through the use of grounding, one can overcome or lessen visual dependence. We do this by using sensory re-weighting. Sensory-re-weighting is a fancy term that means we are training your brain to choose your somatosensory, or "touch" system over your visual sense and unreliable vestibular sense. Through grounding your body will learn to recruit the correct balance system to keep you stable. Of note, you do need to have full sensation of your feet and legs to be successful. Thus, if you suffer from neuropathy of the feet, you may need assistive devices like a cane or walker to help you ground. Let's go through some grounding exercises; they are listed from easiest to hardest.

Sitting Sways – While sitting comfortably, with your feet solid on the floor I want you to purposely move with whatever your brain is feeling. If you are feeling a sense of rocking back and forth, move your weight from left-to-right hip in tempo with what your brain is feeling. Be intentional with your movement, and feel your sit bones accept your weight side to side as you shift. Perform with eyes open x 30 seconds, feeling the control of you wanting to move. Then try to find the middle of your "sits" bones, attempting to find the stillness of your body. Ask yourself, *Am I really moving based on what my body is feeling or am I spinning as my brain is trying to suggest*. If you feel in control of your body, repeat with eyes closed x 30 seconds. If you feel a forward and back or circle motion, just repeat the technique above for those sensations. Just do want your brain is feeling and try to ground yourself out of that false perceived motion.

Clock Exercise – Stand with your feet apart in a corner of your home, close but not touching the wall, and picture your feet as a clock. Your toes will be 12 o'clock, your heels will be 6 o'clock, your left foot will be 9 o'clock, and your right foot will be 3 o'clock. Slowly shift your weight forward to 12 o'clock holding at your maximum safe point for 2 seconds, then slowly and carefully shift your weight backwards to 6 o'clock. Repeat 3 times with eyes open and then when you are ready cautiously attempt eyes closed 3 times. Repeat this for 3 and 9 o'clock. In the end, attempting to find the "middle of your clock" or feet. You will use this strategy in all balance and grounding exercises.

Squats into the Chair – Place a chair up against a wall, and stand in front of that chair. With your weight in your heels, slowly and controlled attempt to sit into the chair. Go as low as you feel comfortable, then stand back up with a focus on feeling your thighs engage, your buttocks squeeze, and core tightens as you stand erect. Intentionally, feel your body lower and lift, with complete control of how you engage your muscles carrying yourself upright. Repeat 5 repetitions with eyes open, and 5 repetitions with eyes closed, as able.

Feet Together – Standing in the corner of your room, place feet together. Cross your arms across your chest and try to stand still keeping your weight in the middle of your feet. If you feel a sway to one side attempt to correct. Try to hold 30 seconds with your eyes open and then try with your eyes closed. If you find this easy, attempt the exercise standing on a foam pad or couch cushion to challenge your ability to ground even more.

Heel-to-Toe Standing – Attempt the same exercise description listed above but stand with your feet in a heel-to-toe stance.

Slow Taps on Step – Stand by your stairs with your hand close to the railing. Slowly lift your leg as if you are marching, barely tap the step in front of you with your toes, and then return the leg down to the ground. Switch to the other leg and repeat 20 repetitions with eyes open.

The exercises listed above are not comprehensive. I work with people on an individual basis trying to tackle what makes them feel unsteady. These exercises are a great start, with the principal purpose of teaching you how to ground no matter what you are doing. These exercises should not make you dizzy. No head movement is involved with these exercises, so the vestibular system is not activated. By keeping the head still, you should not experience any increase in your symptoms. If you do feel an increase in symptoms, it means that your brain does not feel safe and your fight or flight nervous system response is being triggered. To overcome this, use more touch points during your exercises. For example, you can hold a counter or wall for more support until your body trusts that you can keep stable and avoid a fall, and slowly remove your hand support as your balance improves.

We are promoting a very conscious "re-weighting" of the proprioceptive sensory system. The mind-body connection of what you feel, not what you see is the primary focus of all exercises. While performing exercises notice things like how heavy your seat feels in the chair, how supportive the floor feels, where the weight in your foot is being targeted, focus on your and how in control you are of your body. You should aim for completing 20 minutes most days of the week for grounding and balance. You will probably find yourself grounding throughout the day as you walk about. Just try to focus on how steady your feet feel as you walk, and ignore the unreliable visual sense around you and the perceived dizziness in the brain. This will be a large component of our rehab journey. However, it can be exhausting to think about all day; just do what you can!

Nervous System Regulation

The nervous system controls the whole body. It is made up of two systems the parasympathetic and the sympathetic. The sympathetic system is active when the brain perceives a threat, otherwise known as our "fight or flight" response. One may feel symptoms of dizziness, sweaty palms, heart palpitations, or nausea. Alternatively, the parasympathetic system is active when our brain is ready to relax and calm down. The key is a healthy balance of these two systems.

After a person suffers vertigo, the traumatic experience can be stored in the emotional memory centers of the brain, the limbic system. For people suffering from PPPD, the limbic system can experience nearly everything as a threat and can become hypervigilant to even the smallest movements; just anticipating that the dizziness will occur again.

The limbic system has actual links to the vestibular system. This makes for an interesting connection because activation of the vestibular system can trigger a nervous system response causing sweating, dizziness, nausea, clamminess, and palpitations. Alternatively, if the sympathetic nervous system is always "turned on," this will lead to dizziness by stimulating the vestibular system. The solution is, learning how to regulate the nervous system. You want to be able to shut off the fight-or-flight response and engage your calming parasympathetic nervous system whenever you experience dizziness. The following five strategies are tools that you can pull from to start regulating your nervous system. Feel free to explore and find your favorite tool or a combination of techniques! You will want to perform a minimum of five minutes of one of these techniques each day.

Meditation

Meditation is a useful tool that you can use to stop the constant negative cycle of fight or flight in your body. It is a practice that promotes integrating the mind and body to promote a sense of calm. With increased practice meditation has been shown to improve mental clarity, help regulate emotions, reduce stress, decrease anxiety, decrease blood pressure, and improve sleep quality.

To start meditating, set a timer for your intended time frame. Find a safe and comfortable space where you feel supported. You can lie down on the floor, sit in your favorite chair, or simply stand tall- feeling in control of your body. Keep the lights on or off, whatever makes you most comfortable. Feel free to add a weighted blanket to your practice if that makes you feel more grounded and in tune with your body. Choose a sensation, sound, visual image, or phrase to focus on. Stay focused on your body, sound, or mantra throughout your meditation. Try not to make judgments about your thoughts. If your focus slips, just slowly come back to your task and continue through the duration of your meditation.

Here are some helpful links and apps that can further guide your meditation practice.

- **Headspace:** www.headspace.com
- **The Mindfulness App:** www.themindfulnessapp.com
- **Calm:** www.calm.com/app/meditate
- **Insight Timer:** https://insighttimer.com

Breathing Techniques

Breathing exercises are a great technique to calm anxiety and distract from dizziness. These techniques stimulate the vagus nerve, which helps manage the fight-or-flight response and can be used throughout the day. The benefits of incorporating breathing exercises into your practice include:

1) Decreased muscle tension

2) Improved respiration

3) Decrease anxiety

4) Improved sleep

5) Lower blood pressure

6) Lower heart rate

7) Reduction of stress

Here are some of my favorite breathing techniques:

Diaphragmatic Breathing

Diaphragmatic breathing, commonly referred to as belly breathing, is a technique widely used in the medical community to support proper respiration and stress reduction. Here is how you should perform this technique.

Perform comfortably seated or lying down.

Place one hand on your chest and the other just below your ribcage on your stomach.

Slowly breathe in through your nose, feeling your hand and abdomen rise together while keeping your chest relatively still.

Next, purse your lips and exhale as you feel your stomach sink in towards your spine.

Repeat this for up to five to ten minutes for maximum effect.

Alternating Nostril Breathing

Alternate nostril breathing is a simple breathing technique that is often used to calm anxieties.

- To practice alternate nostril breathing, sit in an upright position with a good posture that opens up your chest.
- Use your thumb to close the right-hand nostril and inhale slowly through only your left nostril.
- Pinch your nose closed by bringing your ring finger to your left nostril. Temporarily hold your breath.
- Open up your right nostril by removing your thumb and exhale.
- Hold for a moment before inhaling again through the right nostril.
- Pinch your nose closed again and hold your breath for a moment.
- Now open up the left nostril and exhale. Again, wait a moment before you inhale.

That is one cycle of alternate nostril breathing, which can take up to a minute. Repeat the process for about five to ten minutes or until you feel calm.

4-7-8 Technique

This is my favorite breathing technique! I find it to be perfectly distracting but easy to perform. To perform, find a comfortable place to sit.

Inhale to the count of four

Hold your breath for seven seconds.

- Exhale to the count of eight.

Relaxing breath is the perfect pre-bedtime breathing technique, reducing feelings of tension and anxiety to help you get a better night's sleep. However, you can use any of these techniques throughout the day as needed to quiet your sympathetic nervous system and trigger your calming parasympathetic system.

Tapping

EFT (Emotional Freedom Techniques) or "Tapping" is a body/mind self-help method. Similar to acupuncture it combines a gentle tapping of meridians with mindful and vocal attention to thoughts and feelings. EFT involves tapping with our fingertips on acupuncture points on the hands, face, and body while focusing (temporarily) upon an issue we wish to resolve. The thought is that you can restore energy balance and relieve symptoms a negative experience or emotion may have caused[5].

EFT tapping can be divided into five steps. If you have more than one issue or fear, you can repeat this sequence to address it and reduce or eliminate the intensity of your negative feelings.

1. Identify the issue

For this technique to be effective, you must first identify the issue or fear you have. For many of you, your issue will be vertigo or dizziness. This will be your focal point while you're tapping. Focusing on only one problem at a time is purported to enhance your outcome.

2. Pre-test

After you identify your problem area, you need to identify the intensity of your current symptoms on a 0-10/10 scale. The scale assesses the emotional or physical pain and discomfort you feel from your issue.

3. The set-up

Prior to tapping, you need to establish a phrase that explains what you're trying to address. It must focus on two main goals:

- acknowledging the issues
- accepting yourself despite the problem

The common setup phrase is: "Even though I have this dizziness, I deeply and completely accept myself." You have to focus on how the problem makes you feel to relieve the suffering it causes.

4. EFT tapping sequence

Begin by tapping the side of the hand point while saying your setup phrase three times. Then, tap each following point seven times, moving down the body in this ascending order:

- side of the hand
- top of the head
- eyebrow
- side of the eye
- under the eye
- under the nose
- chin
- beginning of the collarbone
- under the arm

After tapping the underarm point, finish the sequence at the top of the head point.

While tapping the ascending points, recite a reminder phrase to maintain focus on your problem area. If your setup phrase is, "Even though I have this dizziness, I deeply and completely accept myself."

Recite this phrase at each tapping point. Repeat this sequence two or three times.

5. Post Test

At the end of the sequence, rate your intensity level on a scale from 0 to 10. Compare your results with your initial intensity level. You can repeat until you feel you have reached a plateau or are satisfied with the results.

I intend to give you an introduction to EFT as an option for nervous system regulation. This was a generalized explanation of the EFT tapping technique. If you would like to learn more, simply search EFT tapping techniques to find qualified providers in your area who may be able to work with you on an individual basis.

Visualization

Visualization can be a powerful tool when it comes to your future successes and function. Often times my patients have become prisoners to their dizziness and catastrophize every outing they have. They start imagining the worst. The people they will be around, how loud it will be, what kind of food will be served, who they have to talk to, and ready to flee after some self-imposed timeline. That lays the foundation for negative thoughts and negative outcomes. I love to use visualization to form positive neural networks. What if you visualize yourself having a great time at a party? You can just as easily visualize having engaging conversations, being able to get dressed up, having new and interesting foods, and enjoying an evening out! Which visualization approach do you think will lead to better outcomes? Likely the positive mindset!

You can use visualization to start the process of achieving any goal. You can practice visualization to be steady on your feet as you walk. You can visualize shopping at your favorite store, eating at a local restaurant, or taking a beach vacation. When you use visualization for dizziness, it needs to be as specific and real as you can imagine. I want you to picture yourself in a specific place, situation, or state that is positive, confident, and realistic. Over time, visualization can help you see the possibilities of returning to normal function. It decreases the fear associated with tasks or places you have been avoiding and starts to prep the body for what to expect. Thus, positive thoughts will eventually lead to positive outcomes!

Habituation

One key strategy in treating 3PD is habituation. Habituation is a technique that involves repeated exposure to a stimulus until the body becomes accustomed to it and stops reacting negatively. With intentional practice, a person can promote an appropriate response with less anxiety and more confidence by overcoming each specific challenge.

When it comes to dizziness, this means exposing oneself to movements or positions that initially cause dizziness, in a controlled and safe manner, until the body learns to tolerate them without triggering a dizzy response.

This technique can be extremely effective, but it must be done correctly. For habituation to be completely effective, all exercises should truly be individualized and guided. As a vestibular therapist, this workbook will guide you through the process of developing a personalized plan that takes into account your specific triggers and symptoms.

Remember, the goal of habituation is not to avoid the dizziness-inducing stimuli, but rather to gradually expose the body to these stimuli until it no longer reacts with dizziness. This technique can be incredibly powerful in managing PPPD, but it requires patience and persistence.

There are two categories of habituation that I will ask you to perform. The first is known as optokinetic training, and the other is self-movement training. Let's start with discussing optokinetic training.

Optokinetic training is great for people who feel dizzy in busy crowds and environments, like stores or crowds. It is the practice of grounding while watching a video, like a GoPro, in a busy setting. The intention is to focus on your feet or body, noticing what you feel as opposed to what you see in the video. Again, we are trying to habituate you to the busy places that typically trigger your dizziness in a safe comfortable setting at home and asking your brain to pick its "touch" system or its visual system. The practice of optokinetic training can be quite effective in integrating you back into normal community tasks.

Here are the instructions for optokinetic training which you will perform 3-4 days a week:

OptoKinetic Training

- Go to YouTube:
- Search for a GoPro YouTube video of a task that you would like to tackle
- For example, I literally go to the search bar and type in "shopping at Target"

- Start with a small screen, then you can work to a bigger screen, or even virtual reality glasses if you would like

- Only watch one to two videos a day

- Watch 3-5 minutes of any video at one time

- Progression of practice is: started seated, then standing, then standing on a foam pad

- Stop watching the video if you become anxious about it or symptoms increase more than 2-3 points from your baseline starting point

- Close your eyes if you need a break

- Symptoms should return to baseline within 15 minutes

- Watch full screen if you can, audio if you'd like to simulate the store

I also recommend visiting my YouTube page, Treat Dizziness at Home, as I have a playlist on OptoKinetic training with some of my favorite videos. Over time, you will notice it gets easier to ignore the false visual motion and focus on what your body is feeling to decrease dizziness and imbalance. You will also, take the grounding skills you learned in optokinetic training and use them to practice in actual scenarios like stores and restaurants. Thus, leading to your goal of increased function and re-integrating into the community.

Now here is the important part! Each month you are going to be setting goals of what you want to accomplish or have fewer symptoms doing. This is the portion of the workbook that involves setting goals and focusing on getting your function back! It is a crucial portion of your return to health and allows you to pace your recovery according to your capabilities.

Let me give you an example!

Monthly Goals:

1) *I want to stand in the shower with my eyes closed and wash my hair.*

2) *I want to put dishes away without dizziness.*

3) *I want to shop at Target for 30 minutes without dizziness.*

Weekly Goals to Compliment Monthly Goals

1) *Sit in the shower with eyes closed moving head up and down without dizziness for 90 seconds.*

2) *Practice 5 repetitions in each direction of diagonal reaching with controlled head movements and not causing dizziness.*

3) *Practice visualization exercise of shopping through Target 5 minutes a day.*

Daily Tracking of Progress

Monday accomplishments:

List 3 things you did successfully:

1) *Stood 30 seconds and move head up and down twice without dizziness.*

2) *Move head slowly 3 times from bottom to top cabinet with 3/10 dizziness.*

3) *Watched a GoPro of shopping through Target.*

The goal is to take the focus off the symptoms by "reframing the focus". The exercise here is to journal what you have accomplished and your response to an activity. Over time, you will start to reorganize your way of thinking. You will start to appreciate what you can accomplish versus what you cannot. This way of thinking promotes a positive feedback loop for your brain and a sense of accomplishment.

Monthly Goals:

1)_____

2)_____

3)_____

Weekly Goals to Compliment Monthly Goals:

1)_____

2)_____

3)_____

Daily Tracking of Progress:

Monday

1)

2)

3)
Tuesday 1) 2) 3)
Wednesday 1) 2) 3)
Thursday 1) 2) 3)
Friday 1) 2) 3)
Saturday 1)

2)
3)
Sunday 1) 2) 3)

Monthly Goals:

1)_____

2)_____

3)_____

Weekly Goals to Compliment Monthly Goals:

1)_____

2)_____

3)_____

Daily Tracking of Progress:

Monday 1) 2) 3)

Tuesday
1)
2)
3)
Wednesday
1)
2)
3)
Thursday
1)
2)
3)
Friday
1)
2)
3)
Saturday
1)
2)

3)
Sunday
1)
2)
3)

Monthly Goals:

1)_____

2)_____

3)_____

Weekly Goals to Compliment Monthly Goals:

1)_____

2)_____

3)_____

Daily Tracking of Progress:

Monday
1)
2)
3)

Tuesday
1)
2)
3)

Wednesday
1)
2)
3)

Thursday
1)
2)
3)

Friday
1)
2)
3)

Saturday
1)
2)
3)

Sunday
1)
2)
3)

Monthly Goals:

1)_____

2)_____

3)_____

Weekly Goals to Compliment Monthly Goals:

1)_____

2)_____

3)_____

Daily Tracking of Progress:

Monday
1)
2)
3)
Tuesday
1)

2)

3)

Wednesday

1)

2)

3)

Thursday

1)

2)

3)

Friday

1)

2)

3)

Saturday

1)

2)

3)

Sunday

1) 2) 3)

Monthly Goals:

1)_____

2)_____

3)_____

Weekly Goals to Compliment Monthly Goals:

1)_____

2)_____

3)_____

Daily Tracking of Progress:

Monday 1) 2) 3)
Tuesday 1) 2)

3)
Wednesday 1) 2) 3)
Thursday 1) 2) 3)
Friday 1) 2) 3)
Saturday 1) 2) 3)
Sunday 1)

2)
3)

Monthly Goals:

1)_____

2)_____

3)_____

Weekly Goals to Compliment Monthly Goals:

1)_____

2)_____

3)_____

Daily Tracking of Progress:

Monday
1)
2)
3)
Tuesday
1)
2)
3)

Wednesday 1) 2) 3)
Thursday 1) 2) 3)
Friday 1) 2) 3)
Saturday 1) 2) 3)
Sunday 1) 2)

3)

Monthly Goals:

1)_____

2)_____

3)_____

Weekly Goals to Compliment Monthly Goals:

1)_____

2)_____

3)_____

Daily Tracking of Progress:

Monday
1)
2)
3)
Tuesday
1)
2)

3)

Wednesday

1)

2)

3)

Thursday

1)

2)

3)

Friday

1)

2)

3)

Saturday

1)

2)

3)

Sunday

1)

2) 3)

Monthly Goals:

1)_____

2)_____

3)_____

Weekly Goals to Compliment Monthly Goals:

1)_____

2)_____

3)_____

Daily Tracking of Progress:

Monday
1) 2) 3)
Tuesday 1) 2) 3)

Wednesday
1)
2)
3)
Thursday
1)
2)
3)
Friday
1)
2)
3)
Saturday
1)
2)
3)
Sunday
1)
2)

3)

Monthly Goals:

1)_____

2)_____

3)_____

Weekly Goals to Compliment Monthly Goals:

1)_____

2)_____

3)_____

Daily Tracking of Progress:

Monday
1)
2)
3)
Tuesday
1)
2)
3)

Wednesday
1)
2)
3)

Thursday
1)
2)
3)

Friday
1)
2)
3)

Saturday
1)
2)
3)

Sunday
1)
2)
3)

Monthly Goals:

1)_____

2)_____

3)_____

Weekly Goals to Compliment Monthly Goals:

1)_____

2)_____

3)_____

Daily Tracking of Progress:

Monday
1)
2)
3)
Tuesday
1)
2)
3)
Wednesday
1)

2)

3)

Thursday

1)

2)

3)

Friday

1)

2)

3)

Saturday

1)

2)

3)

Sunday

1)

2)

3)

Monthly Goals:

1)_____

2)_____

3)_____

Weekly Goals to Compliment Monthly Goals:

1)_____

2)_____

3)_____

Daily Tracking of Progress:

Monday
1)
2)
3)
Tuesday
1)
2)
3)
Wednesday
1)

2) 3)
Thursday 1) 2) 3)
Friday 1) 2) 3)
Saturday 1) 2) 3)
Sunday 1) 2) 3)

Monthly Goals:

1)_____

2)_____

3)_____

Weekly Goals to Compliment Monthly Goals:

1)_____

2)_____

3)_____

Daily Tracking of Progress:

Monday
1)
2)
3)
Tuesday
1)
2)
3)
Wednesday
1)

2) 3)
Thursday 1) 2) 3)
Friday 1) 2) 3)
Saturday 1) 2) 3)
Sunday 1) 2) 3)

McMillin Method in Action: Stories of Success

The last piece I want to share with you is a couple of patient stories of the hundreds I used my approach. It is important to know that with time and patience, this method is effective in restoring function and reducing symptoms. No one timeline is the same, but with continued practice, you can expect to manage your dizziness and reduce the intensity. Here are a few accounts to demonstrate the healing process with my vestibular therapy approach.

Marie

I met Marie two and a half years after she was diagnosed with vestibular migraines after receiving the Covid-19 vaccine. She had previous damage to the right vestibular nerve and a confirmed right hypofunction in medical diagnostic testing. Marie also had symptoms of constant rocking sensation in the head, worse with moving around, and busy environments, and better when sitting or lying down. Her migraines were being somewhat managed through diet modifications, medication from a neurologist, and stress management.

Despite her medical management plan, she was still having constant symptoms, and could not go to church, drive on highways, shop without rushing out of the store in twenty minutes, or go out to eat with her husband. We set out to tackle her symptoms with the following plan:

- Gaze stability exercises for the vestibular hypofunction. This allowed the brain to use the vestibular system when she was moving throughout the day, and reduce the dizziness experienced with movement.

- Walking twenty minutes a day in total. Starting indoors at home, then working to tolerate outdoor walking, and then finally on the treadmill.

- Habituation exercises to decrease the brain's sensitivity to stimuli and lower the chances of vestibular migraine occurrence. We started by setting one to two small goals a week until accomplished, and then we would pick one to two more. For example, she wanted to drive on the freeway by herself for 40 minutes to go visit her aging parents. We started with a visualization practice of driving the freeway. Then weaned from taking any anxiety medication while her husband drove her. Next, she drove to her parents' home with her husband, but he drove back. After she felt safe, because she had completed the drive so many times with modifications, she felt ready to drive the entire trip. She did this with success and now her body knows there is nothing that will trigger her dizziness so she can complete the trip without fear. If she needs to drive but is having a symptomatic day for some reason, we just set the expectation that she would listen to her body and take her anxiety medication, ask her husband to drive, or choose an alternate day.

The most important point is that you can push yourself to "touch your symptoms" but you should never ignore and escalate your dizziness to the point it triggers your fight-or-flight alarm, causing a negative cycle of "this activity is harmful, so I must avoid". To this day, Marie simply repeats the habituation process whenever she comes across a situation or movement that gives her dizziness. When her body can anticipate, ground, and then desensitize to the situation- the dizziness goes away!

Jeff

Jeff was referred to me in May of 2022 after being diagnosed with headaches and dizziness post-Covid. He contracted Covid in January of 2022 at which time dizziness was a main symptom of his presentation, symptoms subsided for 2 months and then the dizziness returned in May, which was when I was asked to evaluate his symptoms. He had symptoms of being weak in the knees and feeling faint when in large open spaces. Symptoms seem to increase with eyes closed, visually rich environments, trouble driving over bridges, seeing elevation changes, walking into arenas and airports, and walking up the stairs. He also reported trouble walking on the treadmill, feeling off balance and dizzy when finished. Socially, he reported chronic trouble sleeping, being very active in his community, and having high work demands that increased stress at certain times of the year.

Upon evaluation, I found signs of vestibular hypofunction, meaning one vestibular nerve is weaker than the other. This causes dizziness with quick turns, running, closing eyes, imbalance in dark environments, and unsteady surfaces like the treadmill. In addition to the hypofunction, his symptoms of dizziness in busy visual environments suggested a sensory weighting disorder, like 3PD. His feelings of dizziness, when the surroundings were moving without him moving, suggested that his brain chose to prioritize visual input versus his remaining vestibular input or touch system. He also noted an increase in neck tightness and dull headaches, that increased when he was more dizzy.

Over two months, we established a gaze stability program that slowly advanced to walking, added eyes-closed balance exercises, grounding strategies, calming strategies when in busy visual places, and picking new visual challenges for him to desensitize to busy environments in a controlled gradual progression. I also saw him for monthly deep tissue massage sessions focused on the muscles at the base of the skull and upper trap tightness for any neck contribution to his dizziness.

Jeff did well in this program for months. He progressed the gaze stability exercises to the highest level of walking outside. He was able to ground in familiar environments and drive in familiar settings. However, when stressful periods arose or his immune system was down and he got sick the same visually provoked dizziness would intensify. We had to adjust his program to desensitize to more visually complex environments by using YouTube GoPro videos and talking through the process of grounding with hands and feet when he felt overwhelmed by dizziness. I still see Jeff occasionally for neck issues but through vestibular exercises, education, grounding, and balance training he can manage any visually triggering dizzy spells that may arise.

Stephanie

I met Stephanie at the end of 2021. Her onset of vertigo occurred spontaneously eleven years prior and she has been on disability since. As Stephanie, she recounts, "I spent years wandering aimlessly in the medical community only to find myself hopeless, alone, and afraid. My anxiety was through the roof. The medical professionals I've seen were nothing but empty promises and some were downright lies. I had a highly respected ENT tell me all my symptoms were in my head and I needed to see a psychiatrist (exit office bawling) and another functional doc that told me point blank 'I can cure you!' Of course, thousands of dollars later and when that didn't happen, I was once again left devastated."

As you can see, she was quite frustrated and feeling helpless with the various overlapping opinions that left her feeling alone and conflicted about how to manage medical care. She did have a counselor and used meditation and prayer to cope. She had negative testing on brain MRI, inner ear testing, and audiology. Despite all the negative testing, she had constant 4-10/10 dizziness. She was taking daily Meclizine, Zofran, and Ativan to calm her symptoms, but still very little relief. Stephanie was nearly confined to her home. She could not shop, or go out to eat, was not able to do her normal housework, was sleeping 10-11 hours a day, and felt 30% of her normal function. That is when I stepped in.

We started with a plan of cardiovascular exercise using a seated stepper for up to twenty minutes a day. We also added gaze stability exercises and eye tracking exercises to desensitize to visually busy environments; using a very slow pace, one exercise at a time, and seated with full body support. Over time, as she discovered she was safe and in control of her body, we added more repetitions and made the exercises harder by standing or walking. We always made sure to listen to her body and if something felt too anxiety-provoking we would table the activity and think about what we could do to make her feel successful instead.

Then we started with the habituation goal setting. We would choose one or two goals she wanted to tackle. For example, she wanted to be able to shop without her husband. So, we started by examining why she believed she needed to see him while shopping to feel less dizzy and anxious. Then we set a goal for her husband to go shopping with her but leave for 3 minutes, then 5, then 10, and so on until she could shop without him and meet him in the car. The next goal was to drive herself to the store, shop, and return. We followed the process of setting and accomplishing bite-size goals until she was able to drive herself to and from the store. She was able to stop her daily use of Meclizine and Zofran, and only uses them on bad days. She still uses 1 mg of Ativan daily but has the goal of only using this as a rescue drug someday. She can work around the house and ignore the dizziness for many days. Stephanie will tell you she never has a dizzy-free day but her intensity levels are much lower, at a 1-3/10 scale most days.

Again, it can be a very slow process. However, if you follow my process of setting small obtainable goals, celebrating your accomplishments, and continuing to strive for new milestones you will succeed in your journey of overcoming chronic dizziness. Stephanie said it best, "You believed in me and helped me to believe in myself. This therapy process has helped me be more confident. Some days I am able to just ignore my symptoms because of the decrease in severity and improved mindset. You have given me the tools/exercises to help me manage my chronic illness and improve my quality of life and shared with me your knowledge to implement them. All, with most importantly, compassion and commitment."

Current Functional Limitation Tracker

To be used as needed to track progress and current limitations. Make copies as needed for tracking purposes.

Date:_____

My Current Functional Limitations Include:

_____

_____

_____

_____

_____

_____

_____

_____

_____

_____

My Current Symptoms Include:

Please Rank the Intensity of your symptoms (0-10/10) (0 Being None, 10 Being most

Intense)

_____

_____

_____

_____

_____

_____

_____

_____

_____

_____

_____

_____

_____

_____

CONCLUSION

As you approach the conclusion of this workbook, it's essential to acknowledge the significant strides you have made in your journey to overcome chronic dizziness. You have diligently engaged with the cognitive behavioral strategies and vestibular rehabilitation exercises, demonstrating unwavering commitment and resilience. Through your dedication and perseverance, you have cultivated a deeper understanding of the intricate interplay between your thoughts, emotions, and physical well-being.

Remember that the tools and insights provided in this workbook are intended to serve as a foundation for your ongoing self-care and growth. If you need more time, respect your recovery and continue healing as your body allows. While the journey to managing chronic dizziness may present ongoing challenges, you are now equipped with a robust set of skills and coping mechanisms to navigate these hurdles with confidence and grace.

Moving forward, continue to prioritize self-care, cultivating a supportive network, and nurturing a positive mindset. Embrace the lessons you have learned, celebrating each milestone as a testament to your strength and determination. Let the progress you have achieved fuel your motivation to pursue a life filled with balance, vitality, and joy.

As you venture beyond the pages of this workbook, carry with you the understanding that you are more than your challenges. You possess the resilience to face adversity and the capacity to create a life defined by empowerment and well-being. You are not alone in this journey, and your experiences contribute to a growing community of individuals dedicated to overcoming chronic dizziness and reclaiming their sense of self.

May your path ahead be filled with steady steps, inner peace, and a profound sense of accomplishment. You have the power to shape your narrative and live a life guided by strength and determination. Embrace the possibilities that lie ahead, knowing that you can thrive beyond the constraints of chronic dizziness.

Again, additional resources include my YouTube page, *Treat Dizziness at Home,* where I provide video explanations of the topics discussed in this workbook. I also provide one-on-one coaching for people who need additional guidance; you can contact me at treatdizzinessathome@gmail.com. If you have not seen a vestibular therapist in person, I encourage you to visit https://vestibular.org to find a specialist near you.

Wishing you continued success and fulfillment on your path to wellness and vitality.

With heartfelt regards,

Amy McMillin, Vestibular Physical Therapist

APPENDIX 1
GAZE STABILITY READING CHART

A F L B M G

S P E Q V C

R Z X H J D

T O A S J

Y E F U R M

APPENDIX 2

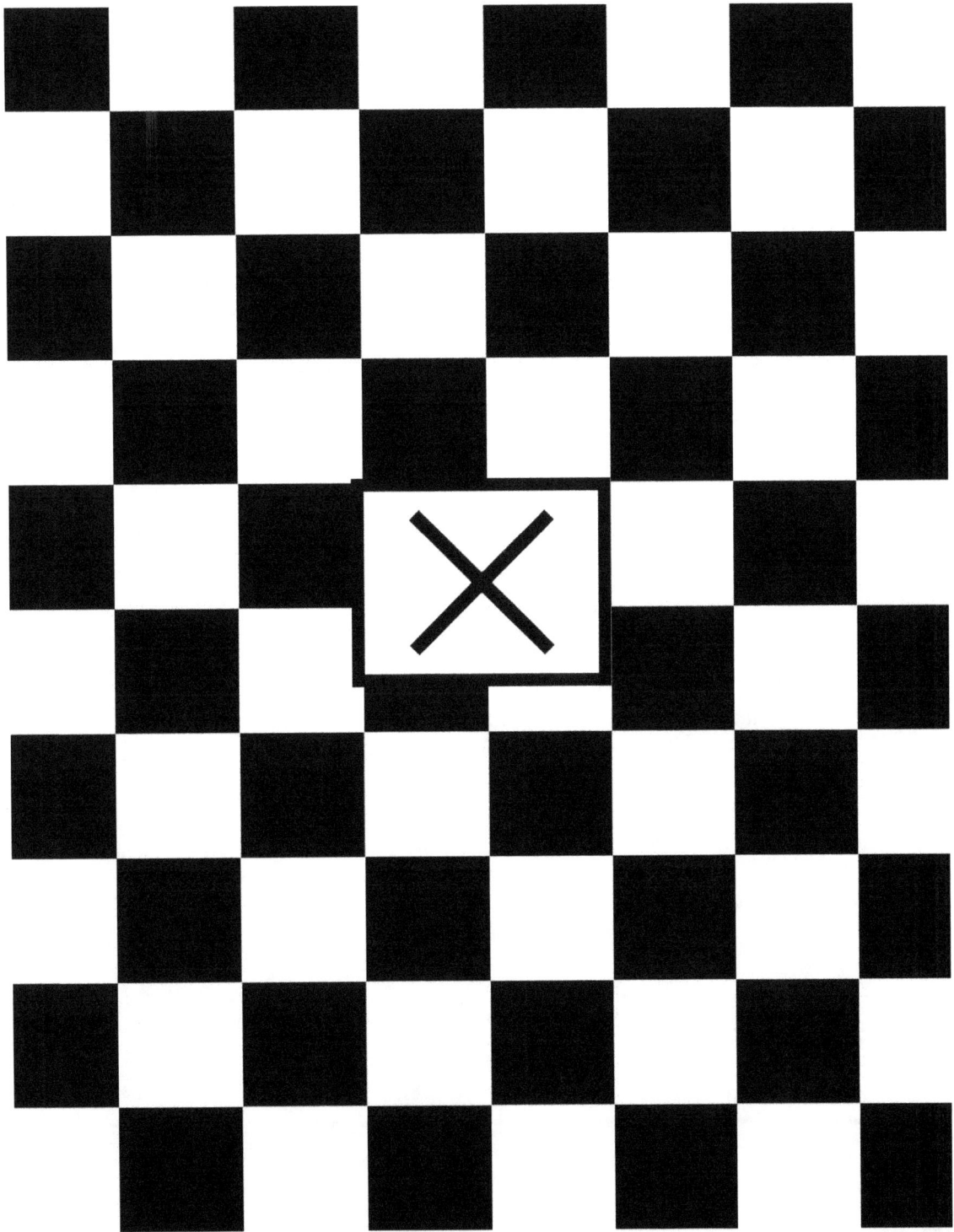

REFERENCES

[1] Brandon Knight, Francisco Bermudez & Carl Shermetaro (2024). *Persistent Postural-Perceptual Dizziness.* Treasure Island, FL: StatPearls Publishing.

[2] *Persistent Postural-Perceptual Dizziness.* Seminars in Neurology. 2020. Doi 10.1055/s-0039-34027362.

[3] Singh, Ben et al. Effectiveness of physical activity interventions for improving depression, anxiety, and distress: an overview of systemic review. British Journal of Sports Medicine. Volume 57, Issue 18, 1203.

[4] Courtney Hall, Susan Herdman, Susan Whitney, Vestibular Rehabilitation for Peripheral Vestibular Hypofunction: An Updated Clinical Practice Guideline from The Academy of Neurologic Physical Therapy of the American Physical Therapy Association. *Journal of Neurologic Physical Therapy* 46(2):p 118-177, April 2022. | *DOI:* 10.1097/NPT.0000000000000382.

[5] König N, Steber S, Seebacher J, et al. *How Therapeutic Tapping Can Alter Neural Correlates of Emotional Prosody Processing in Anxiety.* Brain Sciences. 2019;9(8):206.

www.ingramcontent.com/pod-product-compliance
Lightning Source LLC
Chambersburg PA
CBHW051800200326
41597CB00025B/4631